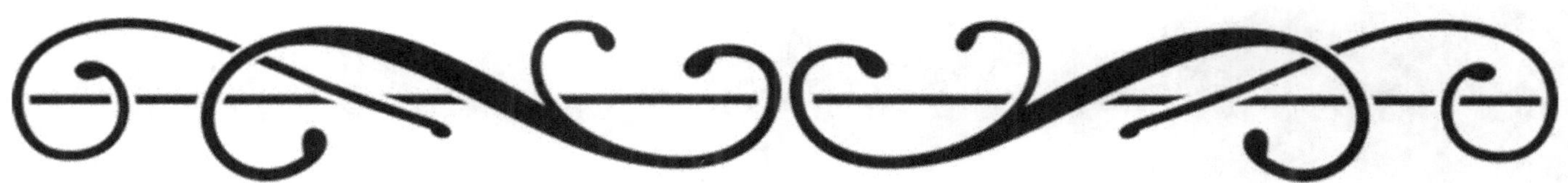

THIS WORKBOOK
Belongs To:

____

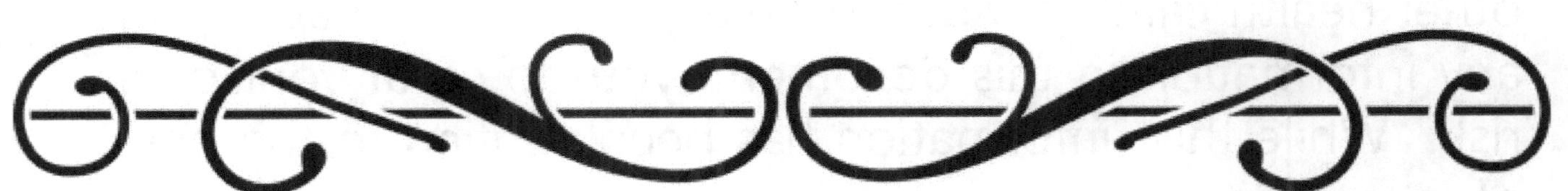

Disclaimer:

All information posted is merely for educational and informational purposes. It is not intended as a substitute for an appropriately qualified and licensed physician or other health care provider. Should you decide to act upon any information in this document, you do so at your own risk. While this information has been verified to the best of our abilities, we cannot guarantee that there are no mistakes or errors.

ALL ABOUT *me*

1. What are you most grateful for in your life?

Keeping track of what you're most grateful for will keep you focused on the blessings in your life. Consider the many reasons you have to be grateful BELOW:

2. What do you love about yourself?

Self love isn't always easy but writing down what you're most proud of will help clear your mind of the criticism and negativity you may feel.

3. Where is your happy place?

Where do you feel most at peace? Do you have a favorite spot that allows you to refocus your energy, find inner peace and feel happiness? Describe your happy place.

ALL ABOUT *me*

4. What do you enjoy doing?

What are your favorite activities where you are able to boost your mood and free your mind? This could be a hobby or physical activity, or perhaps something entirely different.

5. Who can you rely on?

Describe the people in your life that you can count on when things get tough. Who do you feel closest to?

6. How can you improve your life?

What changes can you make that will ultimately improve your life and give you joy? This could be career or personal related. Please share your thoughts below.

ALL ABOUT *me*

7. My greatest accomplishments are:

What are some of the things you are most proud of?

8. What do you wish others knew about you?

What do you wish others knew about who you really are? What do you feel others overlook?

9. What are your greatest aspirations?

Whether it be personal, career or family goals, list them below.

What You Should Know To *Overcome Anxiety*

Learning about anxiety is an important step in the recovery process if you suffer from an anxiety disorder. Anyone who suffers from such a disorder is certainly well versed in the types of symptoms that frequently accompany anxiety attacks; however, in order to learn to cope with and even overcome these symptoms it is imperative that one must first learn why these symptoms occur in connection with anxiety disorders.

The most common symptom of any anxiety disorder is fear itself. This fear often occurs as a result of a perceived threat. In many cases this fear may only result from a threat that is perceived only and not a real threat. This; however, has no effect on the results of the anxiety attack. When the human brains senses fear, whether it is real or perceived only, it responds with certain biological responses. These responses prepare the body to either stay and fight the threat or flee from it. This is commonly known as the fight or flight response.

In most cases anxiety attack symptoms begin to peak within 10 minutes of the attack beginning and the symptoms will begin to subside within a half an hour of the attack starting. In some cases, if severe, it could take several hours for all of the symptoms to completely subside.

In many cases anxiety attacks seem to appear for absolutely no reason. In this regard, they may come completely from out of the blue. Unfortunately, the individual may associate their location at the time of the attack as a cause for the symptoms they experience. As a result they may then begin to avoid that particular location or even situation as a result of fearing the occurrence of another attack. This avoidance can then lead to even further problems such as the development of another disorder known as agoraphobia.

The intensity of the symptoms associated with an anxiety attack can be quite frightening. That intensity level can vary from one person to the next and even from one attack to the next. With that said; however, it is important to understand that while the intensity of these symptoms is often very frightening the symptoms themselves are not dangerous.

Even though the symptoms of an anxiety attack can sometimes feel life-threatening it is important to understand they are not. Understanding and accepting that the symptoms of an anxiety attack will not hurt you is one of the first steps toward recovery. In addition, there are techniques that can be used which will reduce the severity and even the frequency of anxiety attacks.

By taking the time to learn about anxiety attack symptoms you can overcome anxiety disorder.

There are many things you can incorporate into your life to help you to do this and this Planner is about just that!

ANXIETY *debrief*

Describe a situation where you felt anxious:

What were the physical symptoms you experienced?

Did you face the situation or remove yourself from it?

How did you cope with this anxiety? Do you believe your thoughts and reactions were rational?

ANXIETY *levels*

Use the chart below to rate your level of anxiety when facing various situations by coloring the boxes:

SITUATION: Meeting Someone New

ANXIETY LEVEL

DO YOU: Face this fear / Avoid this situation

SITUATION: Going to the grocery store

ANXIETY LEVEL

DO YOU: Face this fear / Avoid this situation

SITUATION: Stating your opinion when potentially controversial or opposing.

ANXIETY LEVEL

DO YOU: Face this fear / Avoid this situation

SITUATION: Stand up for yourself when treated unfairly or poorly.

ANXIETY LEVEL

DO YOU: Face this fear / Avoid this situation

SITUATION: Spending time alone with friends and/or family.

ANXIETY LEVEL

DO YOU: Face this fear / Avoid this situation

SITUATION: Being watched/observed when doing something/completing a task or activity.

ANXIETY LEVEL

DO YOU: Face this fear / Avoid this situation

UNDERSTANDING *anxiety*

Understanding the origin of your anxiety will help you learn new ways to manage your responses.

SITUATION: Meeting Someone New

WHAT IS YOUR BIGGEST FEAR WHEN FACING THIS SITUATION?

SITUATION: Going to the grocery store

WHAT IS YOUR BIGGEST FEAR WHEN FACING THIS SITUATION?

SITUATION: Stating your opinion.

WHAT IS YOUR BIGGEST FEAR WHEN FACING THIS SITUATION?

SITUATION: Stand up for yourself.

WHAT IS YOUR BIGGEST FEAR WHEN FACING THIS SITUATION?

SITUATION: Spending time alone with friends.

WHAT IS YOUR BIGGEST FEAR WHEN FACING THIS SITUATION?

SITUATION: Being watched/observed.

WHAT IS YOUR BIGGEST FEAR WHEN FACING THIS SITUATION?

ANXIETY *Tracker*

Document the days when you experienced anxiety. This page includes a 3-week tracker.

ANXIETY LEVELS (1-MILD, 10 SEVERE)

MON	01	02	03	04	05	06	07	08	09	10	11	12
TUE	01	02	03	04	05	06	07	08	09	10	11	12
WED	01	02	03	04	05	06	07	08	09	10	11	12
THU	01	02	03	04	05	06	07	08	09	10	11	12
FRI	01	02	03	04	05	06	07	08	09	10	11	12
SAT	01	02	03	04	05	06	07	08	09	10	11	12
SUN	01	02	03	04	05	06	07	08	09	10	11	12
MON	01	02	03	04	05	06	07	08	09	10	11	12
TUE	01	02	03	04	05	06	07	08	09	10	11	12
WED	01	02	03	04	05	06	07	08	09	10	11	12
THU	01	02	03	04	05	06	07	08	09	10	11	12
FRI	01	02	03	04	05	06	07	08	09	10	11	12
SAT	01	02	03	04	05	06	07	08	09	10	11	12
SUN	01	02	03	04	05	06	07	08	09	10	11	12
MON	01	02	03	04	05	06	07	08	09	10	11	12
TUE	01	02	03	04	05	06	07	08	09	10	11	12
WED	01	02	03	04	05	06	07	08	09	10	11	12
THU	01	02	03	04	05	06	07	08	09	10	11	12
FRI	01	02	03	04	05	06	07	08	09	10	11	12
SAT	01	02	03	04	05	06	07	08	09	10	11	12
SUN	01	02	03	04	05	06	07	08	09	10	11	12

NOTES:

DATE I STARTED TRACKING:

Practical Steps to Feel Better
and Create Balance

1. Make your life regular like 'clock work.' Go to bed and getup at the same time each day. Give yourself a break today.

2. Say 'No' more often when other people want your time if this is what you feel you need to do. This includes social engagements, the family dinner on Christmas, Thanksgiving etc.

3. Postpone making any changes in your living environment if you have been coping with undue stress. Change of any kind is stressful and limiting it until later is a good strategy if anxiety levels are high.

4. Reduce the number of hours you spend at work or school. If you are a workaholic or school-aholic you need to reduce the energy drain on your body. TAKE SOME TIME OFF.

5. Rest your mind, as mind activities alleviate stress and anxiousness. These mind activities include reading, working on a craft, listening to music, playing a musical instrument, meditation, self-relaxation, dancing or any activity that is relaxing for you. Find something you like to do.

6. Nutritional eating habits and eating small meals helps to keep your blood sugar stabilised. Many people reach for something high in sugar content when feeling stressed or anxious which compounds the problem. Eat more vegetables.

7. Have a worry time if you must worry. When you find yourself worrying over a problem, write it down and then set aside a time to address it e.g. 8pm on Wednesday and then try to park it and put off worrying until that time. Chances are you will not even remember what you were stressing yourself about.

8. Book time for yourself. In your daily or weekly schedule book time first for yourself and then the other activities you are involved in. Don't let anything, except an emergency, usurp your commitment to yourself.

9. Pay really close attention to your levels of self-care, e.g. have a massage or another form of self-care activity.

DEAR FUTURE *Self...*

FAMILY GOALS

CAREER GOALS

SELF CARE

RELATIONSHIP

HEALTH GOALS

FRIENDSHIPS

PERSONAL

FINANCIAL

TRAVEL

PASSIONS

NEW SKILLS

OTHER

5 YEARS FROM NOW

10 YEARS FROM NOW

COPING *Strategies*

Write down the different ways you feel about yourself as well as personal situations, and how you can better manage and cope with self-doubt and negative feelings.

WHEN I'M FEELING...	I WILL MANAGE IT BY...

WHEN I'M FEELING...	I WILL MANAGE IT BY...

WHEN I'M FEELING...	I WILL MANAGE IT BY...

WHEN I'M FEELING...	I WILL MANAGE IT BY...

WHEN I'M FEELING...	I WILL MANAGE IT BY...

WHEN I'M FEELING...	I WILL MANAGE IT BY...

WHEN I'M FEELING...	I WILL MANAGE IT BY...

OTHER IDEAS / NOTES

Living in the Present

A distracted mind is a field where concerns and worries grow easily. Paying attention to what you are doing is key to live a happy and fulfilling life. Having a positive attitude naturally follows.

Decide to get back to the present. For example, if you are washing dishes, start by saying to yourself "this is me washing dishes". Repeat it calmly, focusing on the very act of washing dishes. Name that which you are doing.

As you repeat to yourself "this is me doing (whatever)", you start feeling relaxed. Other matters loose importance; you're giving orders to your mind to actively focus on what you are doing, and only that.

When you move on to the next task, keep on telling yourself what you are doing. "This is me walking upstairs", "this is me feeding the cat", etc. Feel how more and more calm comes to you as you keep on repeating "this is me doing (whatever)".

<u>My Story:</u>

"I used to be a person who worried about imaginary events in the future, and I let my imagination play havoc with me. My worries and my anxiety would not let me focus on whatever I was doing.

Furthermore, I was aware that I was being controlled by my worries and that upset me even more – I would put myself down and say to myself, "What sort of person am I that I'm letting myself be controlled by my imagination?"

Fortunately, I came across some readings that allowed me to see the light. I learnt a few techniques that put me in control of myself straight away. I observed that getting rid of anxiety and worries was not such a difficult task after all.

I am sharing today this powerful technique with you. It is the "This Is Me Doing This" positive technique: getting back to the present (and only the present)".

After a few minutes of keeping focused and repeating to yourself what you are doing, you will probably experience a feeling of well-being. All stresses and worries may seem past or worthless. Keep focused.

Talk to yourself positively in between telling yourself what you are doing. Say "this is me brushing my teeth" (for instance), followed by "I am calm and I am enjoying the present", "this is me brushing my teeth", "I feel good and relaxed".

The benefits of this technique are powerful and almost immediate. It allows you to focus on this present rather than letting your mind play with hypothetical events. It shuts all unnecessary worries and anxieties.

When practised regularly, this technique gives you the chance of being more aware of who you are, where you are, and what you are doing. The very first step to choose the life you want!

SELF AWARENESS *Chart*

It's easy to get lost in our own headspace so it's important that you question any negative feelings so you can sort through your emotions effectively. Use this worksheet to document your progress.

THOUGHT

IS THE THOUGHT VALID?

HOW DO YOU REACT TO THIS NEGATIVE THOUGHT?

WHAT COULD YOU DO TO AVOID FEELING THIS WAY?

THOUGHTS & REFLECTIONS

THOUGHTS *Tracker*

MONDAY'S THOUGHTS

TUESDAY'S THOUGHTS

WEDNESDAY'S THOUGHTS

THURSDAY'S THOUGHTS

FRIDAY'S THOUGHTS

SATURDAY'S THOUGHTS

SUNDAY'S THOUGHTS

TRANSFORMING *Thoughts*

We all deal with negative thoughts and self-doubt. Use this space to keep track of those feelings and focus on how you can replace them with positive thoughts that promote self-growth.

NEGATIVE THOUGHT	REPLACEMENT THOUGHT
NEGATIVE THOUGHT	REPLACEMENT THOUGHT
NEGATIVE THOUGHT	REPLACEMENT THOUGHT
NEGATIVE THOUGHT	REPLACEMENT THOUGHT
NEGATIVE THOUGHT	REPLACEMENT THOUGHT
NEGATIVE THOUGHT	REPLACEMENT THOUGHT

PERSONAL REFLECTIONS

THOUGHT *Log*

Keep track of negative thoughts so you can learn how to control irrational responses and triggers.

DATE	INCIDENT	INITIAL REACTION	RATIONAL REACTION

GRATEFUL *Life*

What are the things you are most grateful for? Spend time self-reflecting on the many blessings in your life. Shift your focus on gratitude and rid yourself of negative emotions and toxic thoughts.

1	2	3
4	5	6
7	8	9
10	11	12

GRATEFUL *Heart*

DAY — TODAY I AM GRATEFUL FOR:

1
2
3
4
5
6
7
8
9
10
11
12
13
14
15
16
17
18
19
20
21
22
23
24
25
26
27
28
29
30
31

Making Happiness a *Choice*

For many people, their personal happiness is not a priority in their life. Too often, we put the happiness of others before our own. While this may please our children, spouse, or boss, this is not the path to happiness. This dos not mean you should make yourself happy at the expense of others, but you must remember that the reverse should also not be true — your happiness should not be sacrificed to make others happy.

Once you have determined to make your pursuit of happiness a priority you need to determine just what it is that makes you happy. Spend some time reviewing the happy times in your life. Think about memories that make you smile or activities that make you joyful. Can you find a common element or theme? Then that is one of the keys to finding true happiness for you.

Now that you have identified what makes you happy you need to engage in that activity. Perhaps you need a creative outlet? Join a writing group, take an art class, or learn an instrument. Do you need physical activity? Then find a way to get back into a sport you love or start a new one. All that is necessary is that you find a way to reconnect with this key element.

However true happiness for most of us is not dependent solely on finding that one key. For most of us, we also require special people in our lives to be happy. Perhaps you have lost touch with someone important and can reach out to them? Or perhaps it is simply a time to plan some special time with family. It is important to our own pursuit of happiness to stay connected with those we love.

Another essential to finding true happiness is to give of ourselves as well. Helping others in both small and large ways can help make you happier and more content. You might even be able to find a way to combine giving and engaging in an activity that makes you happy. For example, if you love to make people laugh you could organize a community talent show as a fundraiser for a local charity.

Finally, make a list of all the aspects of your life that do make you happy. So many of us get down because we dwell on the negative, but usually there is something about your life that makes you happy. Make a list of these items so you can have a quick mood enhancer when you feel down.

The pursuit of happiness does not have to be challenging or arduous. Finding true happiness can be as simply as determining, identifying, engaging, connecting, giving and reminding yourself that Happiness is a choice and only we can make it happen.

HAPPINESS Is...

Complete the following sentences to refocus your mind on the joys in your life:

I FEEL MOST RELAXED WHEN:

I AM LESS STRESSED WHEN:

MY STRENGTHS ARE:

I AM A GOOD FRIEND BECAUSE:

I AM MOST EXCITED BY:

I AM MOST FOCUSED WHEN:

I FEEL MOST APPRECIATED WHEN:

I AM MOST MOTIVATED WHEN:

HAPPINESS *Tracker*

Keep track of how often you feel happy and calm and what you did to minimize negative responses.

DATE:

HAPPINESS RATING: ☆ ☆ ☆ ☆ ☆

DATE:

HAPPINESS RATING: ☆ ☆ ☆ ☆ ☆

DATE:

HAPPINESS RATING: ☆ ☆ ☆ ☆ ☆

DATE:

HAPPINESS RATING: ☆ ☆ ☆ ☆ ☆

DATE:

HAPPINESS RATING: ☆ ☆ ☆ ☆ ☆

DATE:

HAPPINESS RATING: ☆ ☆ ☆ ☆ ☆

MOOD *Chart*

Use the wheel below to document your moods every month.
Use 3 different colors to represent positive, negative or neutral emotions.

POSITIVE   NEGATIVE   NEUTRAL

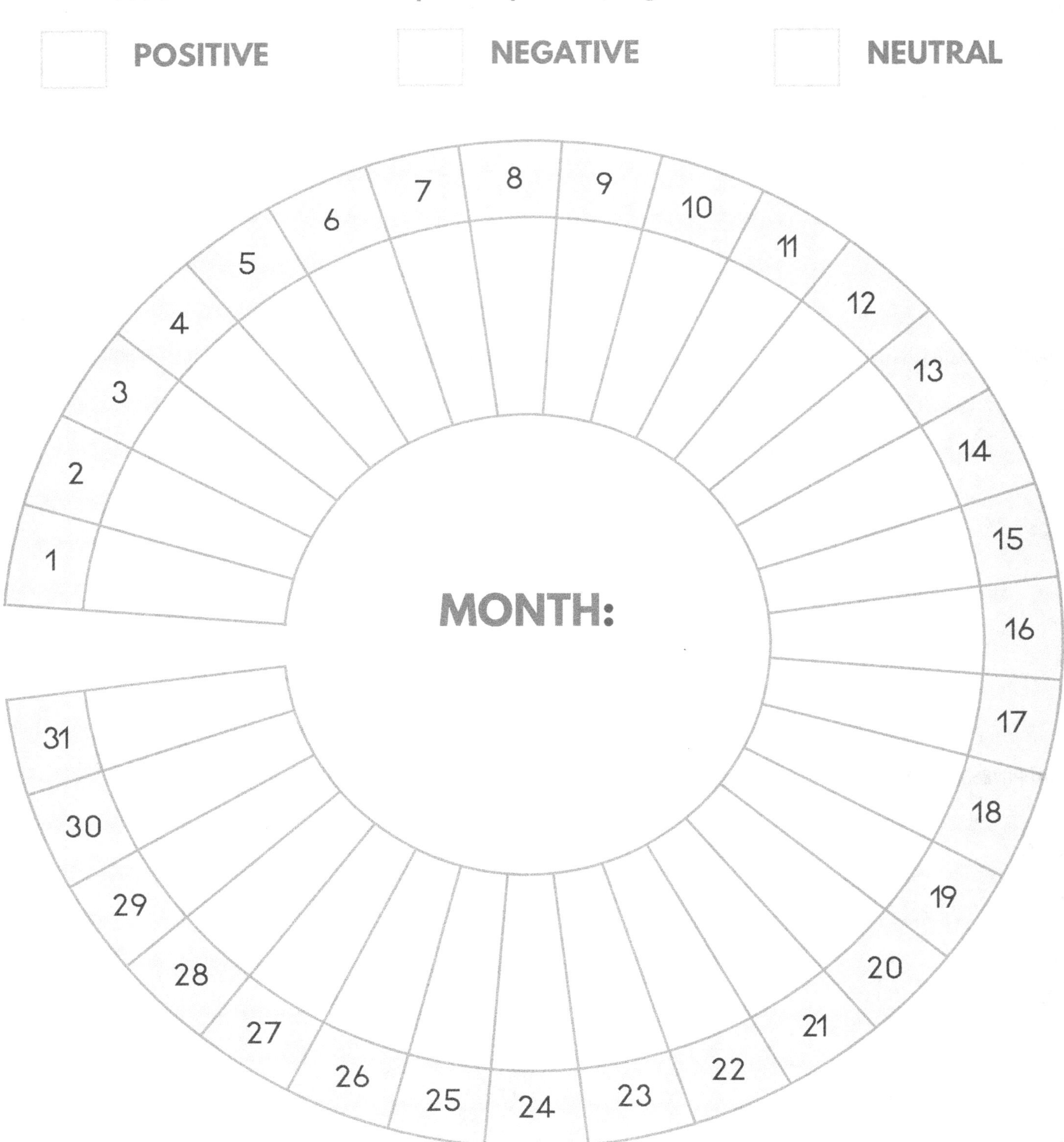

SLEEP *Tracker*

MONTH: _______________

Sleep plays a major factor in our ability to cope with anxiety and depression. Keep track of your sleep pattern in order to determine how the amount of rest may be affecting your mental health.

DAY	HOURS SLEPT	QUALITY OF SLEEP	THOUGHTS
1			
2			
3			
4			
5			
6			
7			
8			
9			
10			
11			
12			
13			
14			
15			
16			
17			
18			
19			
20			
21			
22			
23			
24			
25			
26			
27			
28			
29			
30			
31			

LIFE *Assessment*

TOP 3 AREAS OF YOUR LIFE YOU'D LIKE TO **IMPROVE**

01

02

03

3 WAYS YOU CAN **ACCOMPLISH** YOUR LIFE GOALS

TRIGGER *Tracker*

Keep track of experiences that generate negative thoughts and emotions.

DATE	INCIDENT	REACTION

DAILY *Reflection*

DATE:

HOW I FEEL TODAY

MY GREATEST CHALLENGE

MOOD TRACKER:

MORNING:

EVENING:

I FELT HAPPY WHEN:

I FELT EXCITED WHEN:

I FELT ENERGIZED WHEN:

Today's Highlights

What I'm Grateful For Today

DAILY Awareness

MONTH:

M   T   W   T   F   S   S

☐ ☐ ☐ ☐ ☐ ☐ ☐

HOW I'M FEELING TODAY

3 WORDS TO DESCRIBE MY DAY

STRUGGLES

HIGHLIGHT OF MY DAY

DAILY ACCOMPLISHMENTS

SELF *Improvement*

WHAT ARE YOUR SELF SABOTAGE HABITS?

Eliminate Negative Habits

Create Positive Habits

HOW CAN YOU IMPROVE YOUR MENTAL HEALTH?

What Key Areas Need Work?

What Are Some Steps You Can Take?

ANALYZING THE PEOPLE IN YOUR LIFE

Who Are The Negative Influences?

Who Are The Positive Influences?

HOW DO I HOLD MYSELF ACCOUNTABLE?

What I Know I'm Responsible For

Who Helps Keep Me Accountable?

12 Questions To Assess Your Level of *Self Care*

At some point, you need to ask yourself the difficult questions in order to determine whether you are doing the right thing by *you*. It's up to you to protect your own self from mental health issues, burnouts, and fatigue. Luckily there is an easy way to do so and you can assess whether you are providing yourself with enough self-care by answering just a few questions.

In fairness, your level of self-care will vary depending on the time in your life. Sometimes getting hopefully lost in the woods is the only way to find a new path, for it is in those moments of strife the scales fall from your eyes and you realize how far you have strayed from who you are.

It isn't easy, to be honest with yourself about what changes you need to make in your life, however, the only way to get the best from this exercise is by being brutally honest. We are all guilty of telling ourselves lies, so it's time for openness and honesty.

You may find that some questions hard to face but this is the only way to make changes for an improved life. Even one little step can make a difference. There is no right answer, there are only honest answers that lead to eureka moments. Don't feel shame about your answer – see it as a lightbulb moment.

The 12 Questions

1. Can you make and take time for you without feeling pangs of guilt?
2. Are your leisure activities a priority in your life?
3. Do you understand the difference between self-indulgence and self-care?
4. Do you feel as though you *deserve* your self-care?
5. Do you feel okay about sometimes slowing down?
6. Do you take care of your needs and desires?
7. Do you say yes to requests from others when it is best for you to say no?
8. Do you do things you really don't want to do, or that will over-extend you?
9. Are you running on empty?
10. Are you overwhelmed?
11. Are you chronically tired and have a lack of energy?
12. Do you crave and eat junk food often, and especially during times of stress?

Don't judge yourself or your answers, just allow yourself to be aware of where you are with your needs and wants as well as your general habits and stress levels.

10 Ways To Improve How You Care For Yourself

We all do it. We put our needs on a back burner to take care of work, family, or friends first. It's in our DNA, but doing it repeatedly is suffocating and will slowly suck the life out of you.

But news flash: if you don't take care of yourself, no one else will. It's that simple.

1. Improve your sleep. Make a nightly routine to calm down all the noise from the day, and the adrenaline pumping in your veins. Don't eat heavy meals at least 2 hours before bedtime. Dim the lights and turn off the TV. Getting good sleep will give your body and mind a break from the day's hectic routine. It'll also give you a chance to rejuvenate and get ready for the next day. This strengthens your concentration and memory skills. It also increases your energy level's so you don't feel wiped out by lunch time.

2. Meditate. Relaxing in general improves your outlook on life. You stop making mountains out of molehills and your ability to think logically improves dramatically. It also brings in a sense of optimism into your life. Just by closing your eyes for 2 minutes while focusing on your breathing will do wonders for your physical and mental states..

You can also do yoga or tai chi, which are also considered specific types of meditation, especially if you do it outside where you can be one with nature

3. Talk to family and friends. Research shows that when connecting with others, especially those close to us, our brain releases "happy" hormones, which lower stress and blood pressure levels. It also gives us a sense of bliss and peace, even if it's just talking on the phone for a couple of minutes.

Having that sense of belonging is crucial to a healthy, well-balanced existence. Volunteer work is also great and helps you connect with people. Also, joining a club with your interests or taking a class will offer you similar results, and you'll meet new people while learning something new, so it's a win-win!

4. Read. Pick up a magazine, follow a blog, or sit down for 10 minutes each day to enjoy a good book. Reading allows our minds to do 2 things: 1. Free itself from daily, tiring thoughts that clutter and exhaust us, and;   2) Spark up your imagination. Both of these things are crucial for healthy living.

5. Use this Journal. Set aside 5 minutes each day to write down the day's events and your feelings towards them. If it was a bad day, then writing it down on paper will relieve you of the burden of carrying around all that negative energy and lower your stress levels. If it was a good day, you'll feel a sense of accomplishment and pride when seeing the day's events on paper.

Either way, it's a therapeutic way to get in touch with your inner self. You can also write down your goals to help you stay focused on what you really want out of life.

6. Explore. Schedule it in your calendar so that once a month, or every weekend if you can manage it, you can learn something new about a topic you've been thinking about or learn a new language. The point is there's a wide world around you, filled with exciting and new things you haven't seen or tried before. It'll put things into perspective and give you a chance to see where you fit in. You can think of it as some much-needed "me" time because you get to do something you enjoy.

7. Speak up. Successful and well-balanced people know that if you don't speak up and say what you want and what you don't want, you'll get trampled on.

We're often so afraid of not fitting in or upsetting our loved ones that we don't speak our thoughts and feelings. However, keeping quiet will make you resent those around you first, and then you'll slowly start to resent yourself.

We usually associate speaking up with being rude or selfish, but when done right, saying how you feel is actually very healthy and therapeutic. Moreover, people on the receiving end will appreciate it because it lets them know where they stand. It also shows your confidence and stability. And who doesn't want that in their lives?

8. Eat and drink right. Maintaining a balanced diet where the amount of food you eat equals the amount of energy you burn is necessary to live a long, healthy life. Taking care of your own self requires hard work and discipline, but it quickly becomes a lifestyle when you do it right and make conscious decisions about what types of food and drink you want going into your body.

9. Maintain high self-esteem. Nothing can be more important than how you think and feel about yourself. It helps bring inner stability while reducing attempts of self-sabotage, which we're all guilty of. Enjoying high self-esteem will make you happy in all of your relationships because you're confident in your own skin, and you know exactly what your likes and dislikes are.

Stopping your inner critic takes time and practice, but by using motivational statements, you'll be able to have a more positive outlook. Appreciate everything that makes you YOU and learn how to stop the myth of perfectionism. Instead, focus on your strengths and all you've accomplished in your life - even the small things, because they're part of what makes you special.

10. Surround yourself with supportive people. Sometimes, it's easier to blend in with the crowd and go-with-the-flow. However, that isn't always good for our mental and physical health. We need to have people who know and love us for who we are, without judgment or negativity.

SELF CARE *Ideas*

NURTURE YOUR MIND

Discover new hobbies

Read a book

Take a road trip

Keep a journal

Talk to a friend

Follow inspiring people

Challenge yourself

Be grateful

Call an old friend

Try something new

FEED YOUR SPIRIT

Have "me-time"

Listen to music

Read poetry

Write "future-self"

Paint

Meditate

TAKE CARE OF YOUR BODY

Eat healthy

Start a workout plan

Get enough sleep

Stay hydrated

Yoga

Ideas

SELF CARE *Planner*

Self-care involves taking care of yourself emotionally, mentally and physically.
Create a self-care plan by adding activities to the categories below.

MENTAL SELF-CARE

PHYSICAL SELF-CARE (GET ACTIVE)

EMOTIONAL SELF-CARE

DAILY HABITS (SLEEP, ETC.)

REACH OUT (SOCIALIZE)

SUPPORT NETWORK

OTHER:

SELF CARE *Tracker*

WEEKLY *Assessment*

	SLEEP	MOOD	POSITIVES	NEGATIVES
MONDAY				
TUESDAY				
WEDNESDAY				
THURSDAY				
FRIDAY				
SATURADY				
SUNDAY				

WEEKLY *Reflections*

Monday

Tuesday

Wednesday

Thursday

Friday

Saturday

Sunday

DEPRESSION *Tracker*

Document the days when you experienced depression. This page includes a 3-week tracker.

DEPRESSION LEVELS (1-MILD, 10 SEVERE)

Day												
MON	01	02	03	04	05	06	07	08	09	10	11	12
TUE	01	02	03	04	05	06	07	08	09	10	11	12
WED	01	02	03	04	05	06	07	08	09	10	11	12
THU	01	02	03	04	05	06	07	08	09	10	11	12
FRI	01	02	03	04	05	06	07	08	09	10	11	12
SAT	01	02	03	04	05	06	07	08	09	10	11	12
SUN	01	02	03	04	05	06	07	08	09	10	11	12
MON	01	02	03	04	05	06	07	08	09	10	11	12
TUE	01	02	03	04	05	06	07	08	09	10	11	12
WED	01	02	03	04	05	06	07	08	09	10	11	12
THU	01	02	03	04	05	06	07	08	09	10	11	12
FRI	01	02	03	04	05	06	07	08	09	10	11	12
SAT	01	02	03	04	05	06	07	08	09	10	11	12
SUN	01	02	03	04	05	06	07	08	09	10	11	12
MON	01	02	03	04	05	06	07	08	09	10	11	12
TUE	01	02	03	04	05	06	07	08	09	10	11	12
WED	01	02	03	04	05	06	07	08	09	10	11	12
THU	01	02	03	04	05	06	07	08	09	10	11	12
FRI	01	02	03	04	05	06	07	08	09	10	11	12
SAT	01	02	03	04	05	06	07	08	09	10	11	12
SUN	01	02	03	04	05	06	07	08	09	10	11	12

NOTES:

DATE I STARTED TRACKING:

The Importance of Relaxation

Need to be sold to why you need relaxation in your life? Then let's check this out!

-

Relaxation Improves Your Working Memory

The longer you work at a high intensity, the poorer your working memory becomes. You will find yourself making silly mistakes or getting a little too forgetful for comfort. Even short periods of high stress affect the memory centers of the brain, which is noticeable how forgetful you become when under pressure.

Relaxation: The Ultimate Relief For Your Hectic Life

Do you schedule down time for relaxation in your life? No? Then something seriously needs to change. If you view relaxation as a waste of productivity hours, you have no idea what you're missing.

Not only should relaxation be mandatory, but regularly scheduling breaks for yourself will only improve productivity over the long haul, as you are fully able to dedicate to your work when you resume.

Relaxation Boosts Your immune System

When you lead a busy life, chances are you don't take good care of your health. The result may end up being the exact opposite of what you wanted- sick days that leave you unable to do anything. Luckily, some regularly scheduled time for R&R can offset this. We all have hectic periods of our life, but the important thing is to deprogram.

Relaxation allows cortisol levels to return to baseline, as there are no pressing matters for you to deal with. Chronically high levels of stress and the hormone cortisol may also contribute to the development of Alzheimer's disease over many years, as it is known to have a strong inflammatory component.

Relaxation Restores The Motivation Centers Of The Brain

Do you ever notice how your drive to work decreases significantly after doing it repetitively for a period of time? In fact, under the prolonged influence of stress, the motivation center of the brain becomes desensitized to dopamine, limiting your ability to feel motivated, or experience pleasure.

This also explains why you have no desire to eat and may resign yourself to hopelessness. Luckily, a well-timed break for relaxation will recharge your batteries. Just keep in mind that there is just so much you can handle under pressure everyone has a breaking point- don't wait to find out what yours is.

Relaxation Keeps Your Heart Healthy

People don't appreciate the danger that running a hectic life can pose to your heart, sadly until it is too late. Not taking time off to relax increases your risk of high blood pressure, heart disease and stroke to name a few.

Plus, cortisol results in greater retention of sodium and water, putting the heart and blood vessels under stress to pump and move blood.

Relaxation is well established to reduce blood pressure, decrease your risk of stroke by promoting vasodilation, and decreasing inflammatory processes in blood vessels.

Relaxation Will Keep You Young

Running a hectic life day after day is the surefire recipe to run your down fast. The greater the impact of the hormone's cortisol and adrenalin, the harder and faster your body works to regenerate cells.

Crazy hectic lives create anxiety, cause sleep deprivation, and high stress is manageable up to 3 months, but after that things can go horribly bad. Take the weekends off, or if you can't sleep in at least one day per week. Your immune system will thank you.

This faster turnover of cells causing hastened aging and cuts down your youth. This is why it is important to live while you're young - go on vacations and throw your feet back and just relax. Work will still be there tomorrow waiting for you, so take your time.

RESET *your mind*

We can't always control the way our thoughts but we can learn to transform negative feelings into positive ones and control our reactions and impulses. Use the chart below to start the process.

WHEN I FEEL LIKE:	I WILL TRY TO CONTROL BY REACTIONS BY:

NOTES & REFLECTIONS

DOODLES & SCRIBBLES

SELF CARE *Focus*

TOP 3 SELF-CARE ACTIVITIES

HOW THEY MAKE ME FEEL

OTHER SELF-CARE ACTIVITIES THAT MAKE ME HAPPY

01

02

03

FAVORITE QUOTES/WORDS OF ENCOURAGEMENT

TRIGGER *Sources*

Discover what causes emotional pain and negative thoughts in your life.

Describe the negative reaction/response you would like to overcome:

Consider the aspects of your life below and write down how each category can cause the above trigger.

PERSONAL

PEOPLE

PLACES

SITUATIONS

Think about the different ways you can overcome your triggers when dealing with each category.
How can you better control your reactions and manage frustrating situations?

Wellness Imperative: Finding "Me" Time

 Many of the people on the planet are pre-programmed to take care of *everybody* else before themselves, this is especially true for women or single parents of either sex. It's hard in this day and age when we try to be mother, father, daughter, son , sister, brother, professional, breadwinner, home maker and carer - we feel the pressure every single day.

But we all know how we can be after a couple of nights (or months) of not getting adequate sleep, or how frustrated we get when we don't get even 15 minutes a day to ourselves. Taking time off to do something you enjoy as a means of taking the edge off and releasing the pent-up pressure of your daily responsibilities isn't a luxury - it's a must! Studies show that when you don't prioritize yourself and your needs for, at least, a few minutes each day, you become resentful of those taking up your time and space. Then you start taking it out on them by lashing out, being frustrated all the time as opposed to your usual calm and sweet self.

Taking a breather gives you the opportunity to relax and recharge so you come back with a better ability to carry out your commitments with more clarity and a sense of enjoyment. Learning to be "in the moment" is crucial to your own personal sense of happiness.

This is what those who practice meditation refer to as "practicing mindfulness." It gives you the power to control your emotions and lower your stress levels. When stress levels are low, your perspective on things tends to be more balanced, and positive, you're not angry as much, you're more organized, in control and energetic.

"We're a multitasking society. If we're having a conversation with a friend, we're thinking about the other things we have to get done," says Allison Cohen, a marriage and family therapist in Los Angeles. "Instead, you need to be present in the moment..."

Here are a few tips to remind you how important it is to carve out some time for yourself.

You deserve it.

In order to lower stress levels, we need to stop feeling guilty about leaving the dishes unwashed, leaving the kids to play on their own for a few minutes, or leaving their work at work. So the first step is to consciously make the decision to free up some minutes during the day for *you* - everything (and everyone) else can wait.

You have to build in battery recharge time," says Margaret Moore, co-director of the Institute of Coaching at McLean Hospital/Harvard Medical School. "We're very good at project management in our work lives, but not so well in our personal lives. Treat it like any project..."

Decide how you'd like to spend these precious minutes.
 Some people exercise, others read a book; some do yoga, some run, while there are those who just want a cup of coffee and some quiet. Whatever provides you with relaxation and a chance to free your thoughts and release some of the pressure, then that's what you should do.

Remember, though, that you should treat this time as you would any other appointment and don't get bullied by your sense of guilt into doing work or running errands during your special time.

It takes practice, but you'll quickly discover that you become a much calmer version of you when you make time for yourself, and who doesn't want that!

Practice smart time management skills.
Whether it's scanning emails, surfing the net or answering personal calls during your workday, then it's time to put a stop to anything that wastes time and leads to nothing. Learning to organize your responsibilities should be your top priority, this will eliminate stress and free up time, which you can use for something more enjoyable.

You can even sit down during the weekend to organize your time and write down everything that should be accomplished for that week. Sometimes, this means that there may be times when you have to say "no" to some obligation or other that you don't want to participate in that doesn't bring satisfaction or joy into your life.

.

On the plus side, if you're facing a problem at work or at home, sometimes the best way to find an answer is to stop thinking about it altogether.

Channel your energy into doing something creative. Being creative could be what you need to grease those brainstorming wheels and regain your focus. It could also be the exact thing you need for better sleep.

Find the time.

 Well, unfortunately, there are only so many hours in a day - you won't ever be able to change that. However, what you can do is free up some time here and there to your own personal gain. Juggling your work or study schedule, traffic and everything in between can be freakishly difficult to handle.

However, all you need are some smart organizational skills, and you can be the one in control of your time, and not the other way around.

 If you drive, use this time to listen to music or the radio. You can even enjoy the quiet and your own thoughts.

- If you can ditch your car and use public transportation, then you can use that time to do something you enjoy, like read a book or writing or even meditation.

- If you can walk, all the better. This way, you're doing some exercising; you can listen to music or an audio book.

- If you have an appointment, try to get there 15 minutes, or even more, early so you can have those minutes to yourself.

- If you can, have lunch by yourself at least once a week. Go to the park to get a break from all noise pollution, or if you can't, stay in your car or a quiet cafe or restaurant where you won't find any distractions. Many associate being alone with loneliness, which couldn't be farther from the truth. Being by yourself allows you to enjoy your own company. You get back in touch with your interests, likes and dislikes so you know exactly what makes you happy, and a stronger version of yourself.

"Solitary time can help you have a better understanding of yourself, your thoughts, and your emotions," says Katherine L. Muller, PsyD, associate director at Center for Integrative Psychotherapy

PERSONAL *Wins*
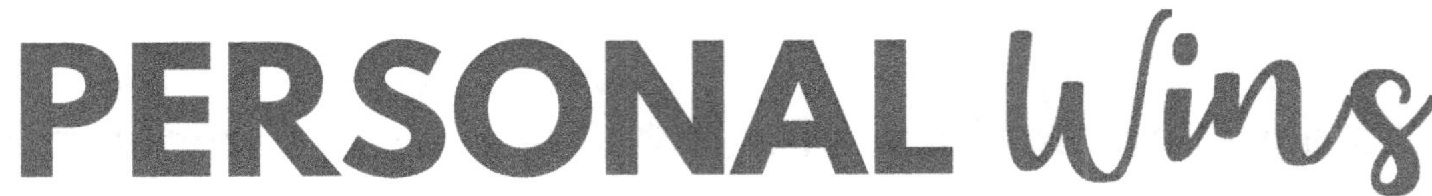

MONTH:

It's important to celebrate both minor and major wins when it comes to your mental health and the coping strategies you've learned along the way. You've come a long way!

2 RECENT WINS

TOP 3 MILESTONES

1

2

3

3 THINGS I'VE LEARNED ABOUT MYSELF OVER THE LAST YEAR

PERSONAL REFLECTIONS

HOW I'VE LEARNED TO COPE WITH EMOTIONS

NOTES

PERSONAL *Rewards*

MONTH:

Make sure to reward yourself for accomplishments throughout your journey.
Whether it's a visit to your favorite restaurant, a bubble bath or an evening with friends, it's important to celebrate your progress every step of the way.

IDEAS FOR PERSONAL REWARDS

1	2
3	4
5	6

HOW I FELT BEFORE	HOW I REWARDED MYSELF	HOW I FELT AFTER REWARD

NOTES	PERSONAL REFLECTIONS/THOUGHTS

LOVE *Yourself*

STEP 1: MAKE YOURSELF A PRIORITY

It's important to always put yourself first by listening to your inner voice. Let it guide you in eliminating toxic people and negative sources. Don't be afraid to distance yourself from people and places that make you feel unhappy or who don't support your journey.

STEP 2: FACE YOUR FEARS

Don't be afraid to confront your fears and self-doubt. Why do you feel unworthy at times? What are you most worried about?

STEP 3: BE ACCOUNTABLE

Hold yourself accountable for the things you can control and change. There are things in your life only you can change.

STEP 4: FORGIVE YOURSELF

Let go of past mistakes – you can't go back in time. We all have regrets and while it's important to hold yourself accountable for mistakes, you can only truly heal when you learn to forgive yourself. Free your mind so it can focus on a better you and a happier tomorrow.

STEP 5: ACCEPT WHERE YOU ARE IN YOUR JOURNEY

Don't allow yourself to grow frustrated that you aren't able to race towards the finish line. Your journey will take time so give yourself permission to fail while also learning to accept where you are right now. Take it one day at a time. You owe it to yourself to stay focused on the road ahead while celebrating every milestone along the way.

Write down your thoughts, reflections and ideas below:

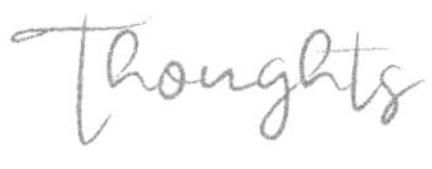